Whispers of the Soul
Finding Hope and Healing in Life's Darkest Moments

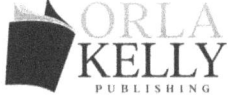

Evelyn Mannion

978-1-917728-25-6

Copyright © Evelyn Mannion 2025

All rights reserved.

All intellectual property rights, including copyright, design rights, and publishing rights, rest with the author. No part of this book may be reproduced or transmitted in any way, including any written, electronic, recording, or photocopying, without written permission of the author. The content of this book is for informational purposes only and is not intended to diagnose, treat, cure, or prevent any condition or disease. You understand that this book is not intended as a substitute for consultation with a licensed practitioner. Views expressed are the author's own based on their experience as a holistic therapist and as a qualified practitioner in Bioenergy Healing, Reiki, and EFT Tapping. Published in Ireland by Orla Kelly Publishing, Cork.

Orla Kelly Publishing
27 Kilbrody
Mount Oval,
Rochestown
Cork,
Ireland.

About the Author

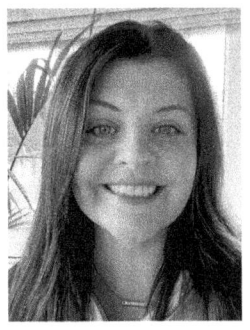

Evelyn Mannion is a compassionate and deeply intuitive holistic therapist based in Athlone, Ireland (eriuenergyhealing.com). With qualifications in Bioenergy Healing, Reiki, and EFT Tapping, Evelyn specialises in guiding individuals through grief, emotional overwhelm, and loss. Her practice is rooted in empathy and understanding after experiencing profound personal losses, including the death of her father, a miscarriage and the emotional challenges of motherhood. These personal journeys shaped her healing approach where she turned inward to heal, rediscovering herself through meditation, journaling, and connection with the Divine.

Through workshops, retreats, and one-on-one sessions, Evelyn gently guides others through their own emotional and spiritual healing journeys, creating nurturing spaces for others to reconnect with their inner light. Her mission is clear: to remind everyone, no matter how lost they feel, that healing, growth, and hope are always within reach and that even in our darkest moments, we are never alone.

Her debut book, *Whispers of the Soul*, is both a heartfelt reflection and a practical guide for those feeling unable to move forward, no matter how much healing they have tried. With tools such as guided meditations and journaling prompts, Evelyn offers pathways towards transformation, ensuring her readers feel seen and supported.

Contents

About the Author iii
Who this Book is For vii
Introduction: Whispers of the Soul 1
Chapter 1: Grace and Grief 3
Chapter 2: Whispers from Within 6
Chapter 3: The Lost Child's Return 10
Chapter 4: She Who Was Always There 18
Chapter 5: Whispers from My Ancestors 24
Chapter 6: The Power of Feeling 31
Chapter 7: The Art of Letting Go 36
Chapter 8: Returning to Wholeness 40
Chapter 9: Coming Home to Myself 44
Chapter 10: The Divine in the Everyday 47
Chapter 11: The Gift of Motherhood – My Why 54
Chapter 12: Never Alone – Wings of Light 60
Chapter 13: Whispers of the Divine 64
Epilogue: And so, I Whisper Back 66
Next Steps 70

WHO THIS BOOK IS FOR

Navigating Grief

This book is for you if you are currently dealing with profound loss, whether it be from the death of a loved one, a miscarriage, or another life-altering event and are seeking understanding, solace, and tools to help process these emotions. If you feel overwhelmed by the mental and physical toll of grief and sense a deeper, unresolved layer of pain holding you back from healing, this book is for you.

New Mothers

New mothers transitioning into motherhood can find themselves overwhelmed by the realities of balancing societal expectations with personal challenges will also benefit from this book. Mothers experiencing feelings of isolation, shame, or guilt, particularly when their reality doesn't align with the idealised image of motherhood and who are searching for community, guidance, and reassurance that they are not alone in their struggles.

Healing Practitioners

Healing professionals, including therapists and counsellors, who want to enhance their practice and feel limited by a lack of resources or techniques. Who are searching for practical methods to integrate deeper healing approaches into their work, particularly focusing on areas such as inner child work, ancestral healing, or addressing complex layers of trauma in their clients.

Key Pain Points Addressed
1. **Coping with Grief**: Managing the emotional, mental, and physical toll of loss and finding a sense of hope again.
2. **Feeling Stuck**: A sense that unresolved ancestral or inner wounds are blocking the healing process.
3. **Balancing Motherhood**: Overcoming feelings of guilt, isolation, or shame tied to the pressures of societal norms.
4. **Access to Resources**: Practitioners in need of practical techniques to support clients with deeply rooted trauma.

What You Will Gain
- **Practical Healing Tools**: Journaling techniques, guided meditations, and visualisations to aid emotional release and self-awareness.
- **Understanding of Ancestral Healing**: Clear insights into how inherited trauma affects individuals and how small, intentional efforts can unlock transformation.
- **Empathy and Connection**: Through Evelyn Mannion's raw honesty and relatable storytelling, you will feel emotionally supported and understood.
- **Hope and Empowerment**: A reinforced belief that healing is not only possible but achievable at a deep, lasting level.

INTRODUCTION

Whispers of the Soul

There are moments in life when everything changes in an instant. Moments when time slows, the world becomes unfamiliar, and you are no longer who you once were. For me, that moment came in 2017, when my dad passed away. I was a new mother, cradling my seven-month-old daughter Grace, and yet I felt like a lost child myself. Grieving, aching, and unsure of how to carry the weight of such loss while still holding my baby in my arms.

Exactly one year later, on the anniversary of his death, I miscarried our second baby.

Grief came like a storm, sudden, relentless, and all-consuming. It cracked me open in ways I never imagined. But in those broken places, light began to find its way in. Slowly, painfully, beautifully, I was called inward, to the stillness, to God, and to the whispering truth of my soul.

This book is the story of that journey. It is a love letter to the woman I was, the woman I am becoming, and to anyone who has ever felt lost in the darkness and longed for light. It's about the messiness of healing, the quiet power of feminine energy, the grace of motherhood, and the resilience of the human spirit.

Evelyn Mannion

I write this now as a mother of three beautiful children, Grace, Katie, and Joseph, and the wife of my childhood sweetheart, Sean. Life is full and vibrant again, not because it returned to what it was, but because it became something new, something sacred.

If you are walking through grief, struggling to make sense of your pain, or simply yearning to reconnect with yourself and something greater, I hope my story helps you feel less alone. I hope it reminds you that healing is possible, and that sometimes, the soul whispers its way back to life.

This is *Whispers of the Soul*.

CHAPTER 1

Grace and Grief

When I held my daughter Grace for the first time, time stood still.

She was so tiny, so new, so perfect. Her little chest rising and falling against mine felt like the rhythm of life itself, steady, fragile, miraculous. In that moment, I didn't know that only months later, I'd be navigating the deepest grief I had ever known.

My dad had been diagnosed with lung cancer in March 2016. From the moment we heard the words, something inside me changed. A quiet knowing settled in; this chapter of our lives would be different. We all tried to stay hopeful, to be strong for him, but there was a shadow always hovering just behind us. Even though we knew he was sick, we didn't realise it would happen so soon. There's something about love that clings to time, always believing there will be more.

He passed away when Grace was just seven months old.

I was a new mother, and at the same time, I was grieving the man who raised me. Every day was a tangle of emotions, waking in the night to feed a baby with eyes full of wonder, and walking through the days with a heart heavy from loss. It felt impossible to hold both joy and pain in the same breath, but somehow, I had to.

Grace became my anchor. Her smile, her softness, her need for me pulled me out of bed when all I wanted was to lie curled under the weight of sorrow. And yet, grief was always there. In the lullabies I sang with a lump in my throat. In the conversations I longed to have with him. In the photos that would never be taken, Grandad holding Grace, their faces side by side.

It's a strange thing, to live in the space between beginnings and endings. Grace and grief became my constant companions. One wrapped her fingers around mine. The other wrapped itself around my heart.

That season changed me. It cracked me open and exposed everything I had tucked away. It asked me to slow down, to listen, to feel. And through it all, something deeper began to stir. A quiet whisper that maybe, just maybe, there was a light waiting for me on the other side of all this pain.

Some days, I moved through the motions on autopilot. Feed the baby. Change her. Rock her. Repeat. Other days, I felt everything all at once, the love, the loss, the rage, the softness. I'd find myself crying while folding tiny babygrows or staring out the window with Grace asleep on my chest, wondering how the world was still turning when mine had slowed to a crawl.

I missed my dad terribly. He wasn't just a father, he was a friend, a guide, a gentle presence in my life. I wanted him to see me as a mother. I wanted him to see her. I wanted him to be part of the memories we were just beginning to make. Every first, her first tooth, her first steps, her first giggle, carried a bittersweet ache. I'd catch myself thinking, *Dad would have loved this.*

And then, as if the grief hadn't already taken up enough space in my heart, life dealt us another blow. On the one-year anniversary of his passing, I miscarried our second pregnancy.

There are no words for that kind of pain, the heartbreak of losing a life you've just begun to imagine. It felt cruel. Unfair. Like grief was echoing itself, louder this time, just in case I hadn't been listening. I remember staring at the ceiling one night, empty and hollow, asking, *why, God? Why again?*

But somewhere deep within, a quiet voice began to stir.

It wasn't loud. It wasn't dramatic. It came in whispers, in the still moments between sobs, in the sunlight filtering through the window, in the soft weight of Grace curled up against me. It said, *you are not alone.*

That was the beginning of something sacred. I didn't know it yet, but I had started walking a path back to myself, through the rubble, through the silence, through the deep ache of loss. A path of healing. Of remembering. Of reconnecting with God in a way I had never known before.

I began to notice how grief didn't just break me, it revealed me. It showed me what truly mattered. It softened me in some ways and made me stronger in others. It peeled back the layers I had built to keep myself safe and invited me to live more fully, more honestly, more connected.

Grace and grief shaped me in equal measure. One taught me how to love with my whole being. The other taught me how to hold the love that remains, even when what we love is no longer here.

And in their dance, I started to hear the soul's quiet invitation:

Come closer. Come home.

CHAPTER 2

Whispers from Within

Grief has a strange way of turning the volume down on the outside world, while turning up the whispers from within.

After my father passed, and as I moved through the early days of motherhood, I craved quiet. Not just silence, but stillness. Space to breathe. Space to feel. I began meditating, not to escape, but to be present. I would sit in those quiet spaces with my eyes closed and heart open, imagining my baby in one arm and my father's presence resting beside me. No interruptions. No distractions. Just us.

Meditation became my sanctuary. It was the only time I felt like I could truly *be*, with my grief, with my unborn baby, and with the memory of my dad all at once. There was no need to be strong. No need to hide my tears. Just breath, stillness, and the feeling that maybe, just maybe, I wasn't alone.

That stillness began to open something in me. A softening. A remembering.

Not long after, I found myself drawn to journaling. At first, it was messy and raw. Pages filled with tangled emotions I didn't know how to speak aloud. But slowly, my pen began to guide me somewhere deeper. I wasn't just journaling anymore; I was writing letters to my dad.

"Hi Dad… Grace got her first tooth today."

"Dad, you would've laughed so hard at her first steps, she toddled like she'd had too many drinks!"

"Sometimes I still reach for the phone to call you."

The words poured out like a conversation between souls. A way of keeping him close, of honouring the bond that death could never fully sever. I'd write until I had nothing left to say, and then, when the time felt right, I'd burn the letters. Watching the smoke rise felt like a prayer, a release, and a way of sending my love into the in-between.

In those letters, I began to discover more than memories, I found pieces of myself. My thoughts became clearer. My pain found a voice. And slowly, I began to hear something else, something softer, wiser.

A whisper.

A knowing.

A feeling that deep inside me, I held everything I needed to heal.

In the beginning, meditation was my refuge, a place where I could step out of the noise of daily life and simply be. But as the days turned into weeks, and the weeks into months, something shifted. The quiet moments I carved out for myself no longer felt like an escape; they felt like a return. A return to myself. To my body. To my spirit.

As I settled deeper into my practice, I began to notice more than just the calm. I began to hear what had been buried beneath the surface, whispers of my soul that had been waiting to be heard. They weren't loud, but they were there, steady like a heartbeat.

I realized that in the stillness, I was meeting myself in ways I never had before. I started to feel a sense of connection to something larger than me, something both within and beyond. It was a presence I hadn't expected, a gentle, loving presence that welcomed me with open arms, even when I wasn't sure I could welcome myself.

I began to feel God in the space between my breath, in the quiet of my mind, and in the softness of my heart. The whispers weren't just memories of my dad or the ache of loss. They were invitations. Invitations to heal, to grow, to trust, and to remember who I truly was beneath the layers of grief, fear, and doubt.

Journaling, too, evolved. At first, it was a way to release the heaviness I carried. But over time, it became a practice of communion, not just with my thoughts, but with the divine. The letters to my dad continued, but they shifted from a way of holding on to a way of letting go. The more I wrote, the more I found myself surrendering, not to the grief, but to the process of healing.

I began writing to myself, too. Asking questions. Seeking guidance. Letting the pen flow freely, trusting that whatever words emerged were exactly what I needed to hear. I wrote about my fears, my hopes, my doubts, and my dreams. I wrote about the woman I had been and the woman I was becoming. Slowly, my journal became a sacred space where I could speak to the parts of me, I had ignored or abandoned, my inner child, my feminine energy, my soul.

I wrote letters to her, too.

"Dear little me, I see you. I hear you. I am here to protect you."

"Dear woman within, I trust you. I trust your strength."

As I poured my heart into those pages, I began to feel a quiet shift. I was no longer just processing grief. I was reconnecting with parts of myself that had been lost or buried for years. My inner child, the one who had felt unloved, unseen, and unworthy, began to heal in the safety of my words. My feminine energy, once suppressed by fear and shame, began to rise, full of grace and power.

Through meditation and journaling, I started to witness the unspoken truths that had been locked inside me. I began to understand that my healing wasn't just about moving past the pain; it was about integrating it, embracing it, and allowing it to transform me into someone new. Someone whole.

And slowly, the whispers became louder. The messages clearer. I began to hear the truth: *You are enough. You are loved. You are worthy of peace.*

CHAPTER 3

The Lost Child's Return

My earliest memory of fear began when I was just six years old. It wasn't a fear of the dark or a fear of monsters under the bed, it was a deep, gut-wrenching uncertainty that came when my older sister had a terrible bicycle accident. The chaos that followed is still vivid in my mind. I remember the horror of not knowing what was happening, the panic of seeing my sister's bloodied face, and the sense of helplessness that filled the room. But what affected me the most was the uncertainty. The complete loss of control, not just over the situation, but over my own emotions.

In the days that followed, I was sent away to live with my mother's friend in the Curragh, Co Kildare. At the time, I convinced myself it was like a holiday, masking how I truly felt. The reality, however, was far different. My six-year-old heart and mind couldn't process the fear, the sadness, or the helplessness. I was terrified. I was separated from my family, from my mother, and from my protectors, my dad and my big brother. I missed them all deeply, but I couldn't express it. I couldn't let anyone know how scared I was, because I instinctively knew my mother was overwhelmed, and I didn't want to add to her burden.

So, I buried it.

At that young age, I learned to bury my feelings; to put them out of sight so they wouldn't overwhelm me. I formed the belief that my feelings didn't matter, that the needs of those around me, especially my mother's, were more important than my own.

It's only now, as an adult, that I can look back and see the weight of that moment. It shaped so many aspects of my life without me even realizing it. I carried that belief with me for years, buried beneath layers of other emotions and experiences.

But as I began to heal, I was led back to that six-year-old girl. I began to see her, to feel her fear and sadness. And I realized something important: I had to go back and give her the comfort and validation she never received. I had to tell her that her feelings did matter. I had to tell her that it was okay to be scared, to miss her family, and to feel lost in the chaos of the world around her. I had to let her know that it was okay to be vulnerable.

Through deep inner child work, I went back to that moment, not to relive the trauma, but to heal it. I sat with her in the pain, in the confusion, and I told her that it was okay to feel what she felt. I held her hand in my heart and reassured her that she wasn't alone, that it was okay to express her feelings and that she didn't have to bury them anymore.

As a mother now, I understand the importance of giving my own children the space to express their emotions. I tell them daily that their feelings matter. That it's okay to feel scared, angry, sad, or confused. I make sure they know that their emotions are not burdensome to me, they are a natural part of being human, and I am here to listen, to hold space for them.

One of the best times of day with my kids is when I tuck them in at night. It's not just about the extra few minutes before lights out, it's when they feel the safest, when their little bodies and minds are at rest. It's when they open up, when they share their deepest thoughts and feelings. And I cherish those moments, because I know just how important it is to have someone there who truly listens.

The emotions I buried as a child weren't just locked away, they shaped my beliefs, my relationships, and my sense of self. But now, as an adult, I know that I don't have to keep them buried. I've learned to honour my inner child and to tell her that she matters, that her feelings are valid, and that she doesn't have to carry the weight alone.

As I began to heal my inner child, I found that the journey wasn't linear. There were days when I could access my childhood wounds with love and compassion, and there were days when the pain resurfaced unexpectedly, reminding me of the hurt I had buried for so long. The more I dove into the work of healing, the more I realized that it wasn't just about confronting the past, it was about creating a new narrative, one where I could honour my feelings, my worth, and my voice.

The healing process wasn't just about going back in time; it was about integrating my past self with the woman I had become. I had spent years being "strong" for others, often at the expense of my own needs. But now, I realized that true strength came from vulnerability. It came from giving myself permission to feel, to acknowledge the hurts that had shaped me, and to give myself the love I had so often denied myself.

It wasn't just in meditation or journaling that I began this healing process. It was in every moment that I chose to stop and listen to the voice of my inner child. When my daughter Grace had a tantrum,

I would pause and reflect on the moments when I was a child and felt unheard or unseen. I would remind myself that her feelings were important, even if they seemed small or trivial in the grand scheme of things. I would hold space for her emotions, knowing that, in doing so, I was also healing my own.

As I navigated my own motherhood journey, I came to see just how much of my healing was tied to how I parented. It wasn't just about healing myself, it was about breaking generational patterns and creating a safe space for my children to feel, to express, and to know that their emotions were valid. I had to learn to be the mother I had never fully experienced, one who listened without judgment, one who made sure her children knew they were always enough.

The more I worked through these layers of my past, the more I could see how my childhood had influenced the woman I had become. It wasn't just the trauma of that one moment with my sister's accident that shaped me, it was the sum of all the unspoken moments, the quiet suffering, the buried fears, and the beliefs I had adopted about my own worth.

But in healing my inner child, I didn't just heal myself, I healed the relationships around me. I became more present with my husband, Sean, more able to communicate my needs and fears. I became more patient with my children, more compassionate when they struggled with their emotions. And I began to see my mother with new eyes, recognizing the challenges she had faced and the strength it took for her to keep going. In honouring my inner child, I could honour the inner children in those I loved as well.

Healing my inner child was an act of reclaiming my voice. It was an act of telling my younger self that it was safe to speak, safe to feel, and safe to ask for help. It was about rewriting the stories I had told myself for years, that my emotions were burdensome, that my feelings didn't matter. Through this process, I learned to nurture my inner child, to listen to her, and to create the kind of safety and love I had always longed for.

It was a journey of profound self-discovery, one that revealed the beauty of embracing all parts of myself, even the parts that had once been hidden in shame or fear. And as I healed, I realized that healing wasn't just a personal process, it was a collective one. When we heal ourselves, we heal the world around us. The more I loved and nurtured my inner child, the more I could offer that same love and nurture to those who needed it most.

And so, I made a promise to myself. A promise that I would never again bury my feelings, that I would never again believe that my emotions didn't matter. I would honour my inner child, not just in the quiet moments of meditation and journaling, but in every interaction, every thought, and every choice I made.

In doing so, I would honour the generations before me and the generations to come. I would be the voice that said, "Your feelings matter. You are enough. You are loved."

This was my path to healing. And with each step, I came closer to the woman I was always meant to be, a woman who could love herself fully, without shame, and who could share that love with the world.

If healing your inner child is on your to do list after reading this chapter, please see below some inner child healing prompts to guide you in the right direction.

Prompts for Inner Child Healing

1. **Connect with Your Inner Child**
    - Close your eyes and take a few deep breaths. Imagine yourself at a younger age, perhaps around the same age as when you first experienced a significant emotional event. What does your inner child look like? What is she wearing? Where is she? What does she feel right now? Allow yourself to connect with her in this moment.

2. **Write a Letter to Your Younger Self**
    - Take a moment to write a letter to your inner child. What would you say to her if you could go back and speak to her? What words of comfort or reassurance would you offer her? Let your love flow freely onto the page, without judgment or hesitation.

3. **Acknowledge the Pain**
    - What is one moment from your childhood that you now realize caused you emotional pain? Take a few minutes to reflect on how that moment affected you. What feelings did you bury at the time? How can you honour those feelings now?

4. **Give Your Inner Child Permission to Feel**
    - Think of an emotion that you've often avoided or suppressed. Imagine that your inner child is experiencing

that emotion right now. How can you show her compassion? What message can you give her that it's okay to feel this emotion fully, without shame or guilt?

5. **Create a Safe Space for Your Inner Child**
   - Imagine a safe space for your inner child. It could be a place from your childhood, a cozy room, or a peaceful natural setting. What does it look like? What does it feel like? Spend a few minutes visualizing this space and how you can invite your inner child to come there whenever she feels scared, sad, or overwhelmed.

6. **Healing Affirmations for Your Inner Child**
   - Write or say the following affirmations aloud, allowing them to resonate deep within your soul:
     - *I see you, I hear you, and I honour your feelings.*
     - *You are loved, and you are enough.*
     - *You are safe to express yourself freely and without judgment.*
     - *Your emotions are valid, and you have a voice.*
     - *I am here to take care of you, always.*

7. **Nurturing Your Inner Child**
   - What is one nurturing action you can take today to show your inner child love? Perhaps it's taking time for self-care, allowing yourself to play, or simply sitting with your

feelings. Write down one small way you can nurture your inner child in the coming week.

8. **Visualize Releasing the Past**
    - Sit quietly and take a few deep breaths. Imagine you are holding a small object that represents your pain from the past—a symbol of the wounds you've carried. See yourself gently placing that object in the hands of your inner child, letting her know it's safe to release it. Watch as she releases it into the universe, feeling lighter and more at peace.

CHAPTER 4

She Who Was Always There

There comes a moment on the healing journey when you no longer feel like you're trying to become someone new, instead, you're finally returning home to the version of yourself you were always meant to be. That was what it felt like for me.

After I began reconnecting with my inner child, that frightened, sensitive, sweet six-year-old who just wanted to feel seen and safe, something inside me shifted. The more I held her close, the more my true self began to emerge. Not the version of me that wore strength like a shield, but the one beneath the armour. The one who was soft, intuitive, radiant. The one who felt deeply and loved wildly. The one I had buried, but who had never really left me.

She was still there.

Waiting.

Patiently.

And when I called her back, when I truly welcomed her home, I began to feel whole in a way I didn't even realise I was missing.

This was the part of me that I now recognise as my *feminine energy*. Not in the way the world often defines femininity, appearance, politeness, quiet, but in the truest, most sacred sense. She was fluid, powerful, creative. She was the nurturer and the wild woman, the intuitive guide and the fierce mother. She moved through life slowly, with presence. She trusted herself. She knew her worth. And she didn't need to fight to be seen, she simply *was*.

As I stepped more fully into her, I softened.

But I didn't become weaker.

I became *wiser*.

More attuned.

Freer.

And something beautiful began to happen in my marriage.

Sean and I had been together since we were sixteen. We were childhood sweethearts, best friends who had weathered many storms together, grief, loss, growing pains, and the beautiful, messy chaos of parenthood. For so long, we had been in survival mode, holding it all together, doing our best to make it through each day.

But when I started doing the deep, inner work of healing, something in our relationship began to shift.

As I reclaimed my feminine energy, Sean began to rise in his masculine energy.

It wasn't something we planned or talked about, it just *happened*.

When I stopped trying to control everything, he stepped in more fully as the protector and provider. When I allowed myself to be vulnerable, he rose with strength. When I stopped carrying the weight of the world on my shoulders, he lifted some of it from me and did so gladly.

Our relationship became sacred.

Tender.

Passionate.

Alive.

It was like falling in love all over again, only this time, we weren't teenagers figuring life out. We were a woman and a man, seeing each other clearly for the first time.

For years, I had still viewed Sean through the lens of our youth. He was my boyfriend, the boy I had grown up with. But when I stepped into womanhood, real, grounded womanhood, I saw him differently. I saw the man he had become. Powerful. Solid. Sexy. A man I could trust with my whole heart.

For the first time in our lives together, I didn't feel like I had to *do it all*.

I didn't feel like I had to lead, protect, manage, fix, or hustle to hold everything in place.

Instead, I allowed myself to rest in the safety of his presence.

And let me tell you, there is nothing more magnetic than a woman who is at peace with herself, and nothing more healing than a man who holds space for her with love and reverence.

We found each other again, but in a deeper, more intentional way.

We lit a flame that had been dimmed by years of stress and responsibility.

And in that sacred fire, we danced.

This is the beauty of reclaiming your feminine energy, you don't just reconnect with yourself, you transform your relationships. You allow more softness, more sensuality, more connection, and more presence. You stop performing and start *being*. You stop proving and start *receiving*.

And in that space, you remember:

You were never broken.

You were never lost.

She was always there.

Waiting to rise.

There's a particular moment I often go back to when I think about what it means to feel safe in my feminine energy, and it was during the birth of our daughter, Katie.

I was in labour; the kind that shakes your entire body and makes you question whether you can do it at all. The pain was raw, wild, untamed, but so was I. And yet, through every contraction, every surge of power moving through me, Sean was there. Steady. Calm. Present.

He stood behind me and *held* me, not just physically, but emotionally, energetically. With every wave of pain that passed through me, I leaned into him, and he didn't flinch. He expanded his presence, his masculine energy, and it filled the room. It grounded me. It wrapped around me like a cocoon of safety, and in that space, I surrendered.

I allowed the process to unfold, allowed my body to open, to soften, to bring life into the world.

Not because I wasn't scared, I was. But because I knew I didn't have to be the strong one in that moment. I could collapse into trust, into love, into the arms of a man who was fully embodied in his role as protector.

That's the power of a man in his healthy masculine energy; he doesn't overpower a woman. He *holds* her. He makes space for her to rise, to soften, to open, and to *bloom*.

And in that kind of presence, a woman feels like she can do *anything*.

Even birth a child, in the most natural, painful, and sacred way, without fear swallowing her whole.

I will never forget that moment. Not just because our beautiful daughter entered the world, but because I had never felt so *held*, so *safe*, and so *seen* in my entire life. It was then I realised, this is how the feminine is meant to feel. Not just in labour, but in *life*.

Supported.

Cherished.

Free to let go.

When the masculine is grounded, trustworthy, and loving, the feminine feels safe enough to surrender. And when a woman surrenders, the world changes. Creation happens. Healing happens. *Life* happens.

If this chapter stirred something in you, a longing, a curiosity, or even a sense of grief for what you haven't yet experienced, know that it's not too late. The divine feminine and the sacred masculine live within all of us, and when we begin to honour both, our relationships shift, our hearts soften, and we come home to ourselves. Whether you're in partnership or not, ask yourself: *Where can I let go of control and allow myself to receive? Where can I trust more, soften more, surrender more?* And if you are in a relationship, invite your partner in. Show them the parts of you that long to be held, not fixed. You might be surprised by what blossoms when you allow love to meet you, right where you are.

Journaling Prompts for the divine feminine:

1. *What does it feel like when I am fully in my feminine energy? When was the last time I allowed myself to truly soften, receive, and be held?*
2. *What beliefs do I hold around surrender, vulnerability, or letting someone else support me? Where did those beliefs come from?*
3. *In what ways have I tried to control or carry everything on my own? What would it feel like to lay that burden down?*
4. *How do I perceive the masculine energy in my life — within myself, my partner, or the people around me? Is it something I trust? Why or why not?*
5. *What would it look like for me to invite more balance between the masculine and feminine energies in my daily life, relationships, and spiritual path?*
6. *Write a letter to your feminine self — the woman within you who is longing to be seen, cherished, and free. What does she need to hear right now?*

CHAPTER 5

Whispers from My Ancestors

Who the hell am I?

Where did I come from?

And why do I feel like I've been carrying pain that was never mine to carry?

These were the questions that echoed through me in the quiet moments, before sleep, in the stillness of meditation, or when the overwhelm of motherhood crept in and wrapped itself tightly around me.

Becoming a mother cracked something open.

It was beautiful and raw, and also unbelievably hard.

Some days, with just three little ones, I felt completely outnumbered, like I was being ambushed by tiny, love-filled warriors.

And I found myself thinking of my grandmothers.

How did they do it?

How did they survive motherhood, womanhood, and everything in between, in times when there was no space for softness, no room for self-care or emotional expression?

It was this curiosity, this pull toward the women who came before me, that led me into the world of *ancestral healing*.

For me, ancestral healing was the process of acknowledging, understanding, and transforming the patterns, traumas, and gifts that had been passed down through my lineage, both through blood and through spirit.

I came to understand that our ancestors' unresolved experiences, their grief, their fears, their silence, don't just disappear. They are stored in the body. In the DNA. In the heart.

And if left unspoken, unhealed, they continue through us.

That's when I realised: by healing myself, I wasn't just healing me.

I was healing backwards.

I was healing *them*, the women who never had the chance to speak their truth or rest in their softness.

And I was healing forwards, for my children, and their children still to come.

Heal the past. Free the future.

That became my quiet mantra.

I would look at my kids and feel it so deeply in my bones, *they deserve this*.

And then I'd look at an old photo of my nanny Shine, Tess her name was, and my Granny Leila, whom I never got the opportunity to meet, and whisper, *you deserve this too*.

They didn't have the freedom, the tools, or even the language to do this work.

But I do.

And so, it became not only my responsibility, but my honour.

Despite all the deep healing work I had already done, something still felt stuck. Something lingering, old, and heavy.

It wasn't until I began to explore ancestral energy healing and sacred intention setting, that things began to shift, like truly shift.

I could feel it.

Feel the weight lifting.

Feel the threads unravelling.

It was like my ancestors were whispering, *thank you.*

I imagined them cheering me on.

And I cried.

Because how could I not follow that call?

The truth is, ancestral trauma lives in our nervous systems.

It shows up in our fears, in our sense of being stuck, in the belief that we don't belong, or that we're not safe to be seen.

These wounds are passed down quietly, generation after generation, tucked between family recipes and whispered warnings, in the unsaid things that shaped us more than we realise.

For me, that trauma showed up as a deep-rooted fear, a sense of not belonging, and a heaviness that no amount of rest could relieve.

Once I started to release it, I began to reconnect with my soul in a way I had never known before.

And from that space, deep healing unfolded, for me, for my lineage, and for those yet to come.

Even now, I watch people in my family carry pain that doesn't belong to them, unaware, heavy, hurting.

But healing is a choice.

And while I can't walk the path *for* them, I can stand on the sidelines, with love, and whisper, *when you're ready, I'll be here.*

If you're reading this and feel the call to begin your own ancestral healing journey, I want you to know, you are not alone.

Let this chapter be your first step.

Start with intention.

Start with curiosity.

And start with compassion for yourself and for all who came before you.

You are the cycle breaker.

You are the turning point in your family line.

And your healing is not just for you, it ripples through generations.

❦ *Healing the River of Blood: A Guided Meditation*

As you reflect on the wisdom shared in this chapter, I invite you to pause and take a moment to connect with your ancestors in a deeper, more personal way. Let this guided meditation help you clear ancestral wounds, while also honouring and reclaiming the blessings that have been passed down to you.

Find a quiet space, light a candle, and let yourself be immersed in this healing journey. The path is yours to walk, and the energy of your ancestors will be with you every step of the way.

Step 1: Opening the Space

Place your hands on your heart and take a few deep breaths.

Say aloud or silently:

"I call upon the Light of my Higher Self. I invite in the wisdom and healing of my well ancestors—those who walked before me in love, strength, and truth. I open this space in honour of healing, not blame. May only that which is for my highest good be present here."

Step 2: Grounding

Visualize yourself standing in the middle of a forest. When you look up, you can see the sun sparkling through the thick green leaves of the trees, you can feel a soft breeze and the warmth of the sun, shining down on your face. Feel the security of being held by the cosmic mother. Mother Earth. And visualise roots extending from the base of your spine and feet, anchoring you deep into the Earth.

Feel the Earth holding you. You are safe. You belong here.

Say out loud or in your head:

"I am safe. I am grounded. I am ready."

"I am safe. I am grounded. I am ready."

"I am safe. I am grounded. I am ready."

Step 3: Entering the River of Blood. The river of our lineage.

Close your eyes and imagine yourself standing by a river. You notice some of its waters are clear and beautiful, but also, some are murky and heavy.

Visualise yourself slowly walking into the river. Feel the water as it meets your feet, your legs, and then your waist. As your standing in the river, waist high, you can feel the stories run through every cell of your body, you can hear the laughter and the cries of the past, you can feel the emotions, the strength and the sorrow of your lineage. You can see and you can feel as they are flowing all around you.

Say aloud or silently:

"I stand in the river of those who came before me. I acknowledge the pain they carried. I honour the strength that kept them going. And I choose now to become a vessel of healing—for myself, for them, and for those yet to come. I see you. I hear you. I acknowledge you, but I can't carry what isn't mine any longer. I come here today not to blame but to heal. You deserve healing and so do I."

Step 4: Healing Transmission

Visualize a golden light descending from above, source, spirit, love. Let this golden light flow down into your body and into the river. Watch as the murky waters begin to clear.

You might see faces, memories, or feel emotions, don't block anything, allow whatever arises to be witnessed without judgment.

With each breath, say:

"I release what is not mine to carry."

"I send forgiveness backward through time."

"I carry forward only love, strength, and wisdom."

Step 5: Closing and Offering

Dip your fingers in the bowl of water and sprinkle some around you.

Say:

"With this water, I cleanse the wounds of the past. I bless my body, my soul, and my family line."

Blow out the candle and give thanks to your ancestors, seen and unseen.

Bow your head in silent prayer and begin to journal any insights, emotions, or symbols that came up for you.

Final Reflection:

Ancestral healing is not only about releasing burdens, it's also about *remembering* and *reclaiming* the strength, resilience, and love that have been passed down to you. It's about understanding that your life is part of a bigger story, one that has been unfolding long before you were born.

Now, I encourage you to reflect on what you've experienced during this meditation and any insights that may have arisen. What ancestral patterns or blessings did you encounter? What has been passed down to you that you are ready to release or embrace?

Grab your journal and explore the following prompts:

- What blessings or gifts have you inherited from your ancestors that you feel connected to?
- What are you ready to release, and what will you carry forward with you from your lineage?
- How does healing your ancestral line impact the way you see yourself today?

CHAPTER 6

The Power of Feeling

The Journey to Healing Begins Within

Healing doesn't happen by avoiding discomfort or pushing past painful emotions. In fact, healing begins when we allow ourselves to feel, when we make space for the uncomfortable emotions that are often buried deep within us. In my own journey through grief, I experienced firsthand how suppression of emotion keeps us from healing. I was crying one moment and then pushing myself to move on with the day, not allowing myself to fully process the rawness of my feelings. The anger, the frustration, the deep sadness, these were emotions I didn't know how to handle.

As I continued down this path of avoidance, I realized that I was not honouring how I truly felt. I wasn't letting the emotions pass through me; I was suppressing them. And when emotions are suppressed, they don't go away, they stay within, and they build up. I wasn't allowing myself to grieve fully, to be angry fully, or to be sad. Instead, I tried to carry on as if everything was fine, but this avoidance only made me feel more disconnected from myself.

Sometimes, the most healing thing you can do is sit with discomfort. When we stop pushing the uncomfortable feelings away, when we stop judging ourselves for feeling hurt, grief, or anger, we create the space for those emotions to move through us. It's the simple act of allowing. When we truly feel, we begin to release.

The Body Keeps the Score

If we don't allow ourselves to feel, emotions get stuck. And when emotions remain unexpressed, they can manifest in the body. Suppressed emotions can show up as physical ailments, pain, fatigue, illness, or even disease. It's as though our body is trying to communicate with us, telling us that something is out of alignment.

Our emotions are energy in motion, and when we suppress them, we're essentially blocking that flow. We can only ignore them for so long before they begin to demand attention, often in the form of physical discomfort or even disease. Chronic stress, unresolved grief, and anger that's never expressed can all contribute to various health problems. The body doesn't forget. It stores emotional pain, and over time, that stored pain can manifest in ways we least expect.

I know now that healing is not just a mental or emotional process, it's a holistic one. The emotions we carry are not just memories in our minds; they're energy held in our bodies. When we heal emotionally, we heal physically. The work is not just to clear mental blockages or emotional scars, but to release what has been held in the physical body too.

How to Allow Your Emotions to Move Through You

So, how do we begin to heal? How do we allow those emotions that we've been carrying for so long to finally move through us?

It starts with acknowledgment. You must give yourself permission to feel. Often, the first step is simply recognizing that you are feeling something. Sometimes, this is the hardest part—we're so used to pushing our feelings away that we don't even realize we're holding on to them. But once you acknowledge that you are feeling something, the healing can begin.

Next, we must make space for these emotions. Instead of judging them or labelling them as "bad," we must let them come. Allow yourself to feel sadness, anger, fear, or even joy. You may not be able to control the intensity of the emotion, but you can control how you respond to it. Instead of rejecting the feelings, try welcoming them with compassion.

Allowing yourself to feel is not about indulging in the emotion, but rather, being present with it. You don't have to do anything with it at first, just feel. Let it be there. The more you can let go of the need to control the emotions, the easier they will move through you.

And remember, emotions are temporary. Just as a storm passes, emotions will rise and fall. You do not have to hold on to them forever. The key is to release them when they've moved through you.

Releasing the Emotions: Letting Them Go

Once you've allowed yourself to feel an emotion, the next step is releasing it. You don't have to carry it forever. Often, simply acknowledging and feeling the emotion is enough to allow it to shift. Other times, you may need to actively release it, whether that's through breathwork, journaling, or even a physical activity like shaking, dancing, or moving your body.

This is a practice I've used myself, and I encourage you to try it. When you're feeling overwhelmed by emotion, try placing your hands over your heart and breathing deeply. As you breathe in, acknowledge the emotion. As you breathe out, imagine that emotion leaving your body. Do this until you feel lighter, more peaceful.

Journaling Prompts for Healing

As you work on allowing your emotions to move through you, here are some journaling prompts that can guide you in your healing journey:

1. **What emotions am I holding on to right now?**
2. Write about any feelings that come up, no matter how big or small. Allow yourself to be honest.
3. **When was the last time I allowed myself to truly feel an emotion, without judgment?**
4. Reflect on times when you've held back your feelings. What would have happened if you had let them flow freely?
5. **How does my body feel right now?**
6. Tune into your body. Are there any areas of tension, pain, or discomfort? Write about what those areas might be holding.
7. **What happens when I allow myself to feel my emotions fully?**
8. Reflect on any changes in your mental, emotional, or physical state after you've given yourself the space to feel.
9. **What am I afraid of when I feel my emotions?**
10. Are there any fears or worries about feeling your emotions? Write about what those fears are and see if they hold any truth.

Healing begins when we allow ourselves to feel. It's an act of surrender, not to the emotion, but to the process of releasing. When we sit with our emotions instead of running from them, we allow the healing to flow. By acknowledging what we've been carrying, we free ourselves from the weight of suppression.

Remember, feeling is the first step. It's the necessary foundation for all healing. You don't have to have all the answers right away, but if you can give yourself permission to feel, you've already taken the most important step toward true healing.

CHAPTER 7

The Art of Letting Go

Letting go isn't always about release, it's often about remembering who we are without all the roles we were conditioned to play.

I was the youngest of six children. By the time I came along, my parents had already been through so much, my sister's terrible bike accident, another sister's battle with mental health, and my mother's quiet suffering with depression that seemed to hang like fog over much of my childhood. I made a silent vow early on: *don't be a bother*. I became the "good child," the one who never caused trouble, the one who quietly handled things on her own.

On the surface, I was praised for my independence. Underneath, I was learning to survive by not needing anyone. I didn't know it then, but what I was really doing was building walls, walls of self-sufficiency that made it nearly impossible to ask for help or to trust someone else with my emotions, my decisions, my life.

As I moved through adulthood, this pattern kept showing up. I always felt like I had to carry it all, every emotion, every responsibility, every burden. I lived with an unspoken resentment, an ache that whispered *why didn't anyone hold me?*

But the truth was, I didn't know how to let myself be held.

Letting go of that version of myself, the one who never needed help, who always had it together, was one of the scariest things I've ever done. She had kept me safe. But she was also keeping me from true intimacy, vulnerability, and joy.

Then there was the deep shame I carried after losing my baby. It felt like my body had failed me. I couldn't even speak about it without the energy in the room shifting into discomfort, silence, and avoidance. No one knew what to say. So, I held the grief quietly, almost like a secret, *my dirty little secret*. But healing came the moment I gave myself permission to feel it all, the sorrow, the guilt, the anger. And in doing so, I realised: my body hadn't failed. It had grieved. And it needed me to love it again.

Another layer of letting go came in the form of career. I spent years in jobs I hated, offices, admin work, business roles that made me feel like I was selling my soul to the devil. I stayed because it's what was expected. It was secure. It was "sensible." But it wasn't *me*. Letting go of those expectations, and more importantly, letting go of the version of me that needed to meet them, was the moment life began to bloom.

I stepped into my truth. I trained as a Bio Energy Healing Therapist, an EFT Practitioner, and a Reiki Healing Therapist. I began to serve others through healing. I even found the courage to write this book.

Letting go wasn't the end of me. It was the beginning of everything.

Visualisation: Surrendering into Trust

Find a quiet space and settle into a comfortable seated or lying position. Close your eyes, and take a slow, deep breath in through your nose... and gently sigh it out through your mouth.

Let your body soften.

Let your shoulders drop.

Let your jaw unclench.

Let go of the need to hold it all together for just a few moments.

Now imagine yourself standing in the middle of a beautiful meadow. The grass is tall and golden, dancing gently in the wind. The sky above is open, endless, painted in soft hues of blue and white. The sun is warm on your skin. You are alone, but you are not lonely. You feel safe, held by the stillness around you.

In front of you stands a large hot air balloon, its basket woven with love, its colours vibrant and welcoming. This balloon represents the part of you that is ready to rise. But in your hands, you're holding heavy suitcases, some filled with fear, some with old beliefs, some with the stories that say, *"you must do it all alone."*

One by one, you place the suitcases down beside the balloon. As you release each one, feel your body getting lighter. With every item you set down, whisper to yourself:

"I no longer need to carry this."

You step into the basket. The ropes are untied. The balloon begins to lift. Gently. Peacefully. Without force.

You look down and see all you've let go of. You realise it didn't define you. It never did. And even without it, you are still whole. You are still worthy. You are still you.

Feel the breeze on your face. The freedom. The release. The quiet trust that life is supporting you now.

You don't have to hold it all.

You don't have to know all the answers.

You are safe to surrender.

Stay here for as long as you need, floating in the knowing that when you let go, you make space for the beautiful unknown to arrive.

When you're ready, gently bring your awareness back to your breath... your body... and the space around you. And know this:

You can return here any time you forget how free you really are.

Journaling Prompts for The Art of Letting Go

1. What am I holding onto that no longer serves me?

Reflect on old beliefs, habits, or expectations you may be ready to release.

2. What emotions arise when I think about surrendering control?

Is it fear, grief, relief, or something else? Let them come through without judgment.

3. Where in my life have I felt I had to do it all on my own?

Write about moments or patterns where you carried the weight by yourself—and how that felt in your body.

4. What would it feel like to trust more—myself, others, or life itself?

Explore the idea of leaning into support, softness, and flow.

5. If I could speak to the part of me that's scared to let go, what would I say?

Let this be a loving conversation with your inner self.

6. Where has letting go already brought me more peace or joy?

Sometimes, the proof is already in your story. Honour the growth.

CHAPTER 8

Returning to Wholeness

There's a quiet moment that comes after the release. After the storm of emotions has been felt, honoured, and let go. It doesn't come with fireworks or applause. It comes gently—like a breath you didn't realise you'd been holding, finally exhaled.

That's what returning to wholeness felt like for me.

It wasn't a single moment, but many small ones. Laughing without guilt. Dancing in the kitchen with my kids. Looking in the mirror and actually liking the woman I saw looking back. Whispering "thank you" to the sky without needing anything in return.

I realised that healing isn't about becoming someone new. It's about remembering who I was before the world told me who to be.

Wholeness didn't mean perfection. It meant *integration*. A sacred weaving together of all my parts—the light, the shadow, the mess, the magic. I no longer needed to hide or fix or prove. I was enough. I had always been enough.

And as I returned to myself, I began to trust life again.

I used to think healing was about *fixing* myself. That one day I'd wake up and finally feel "healed", as if pain would no longer exist, and I'd be wrapped in some kind of bubble of perfection.

But real healing… real wholeness… felt more like **coming home.**

It was about learning to trust myself again.

After years of overriding my intuition, second-guessing every decision, and seeking validation outside of me, I began to remember that quiet voice within.

The one that always knew.

Self-trust didn't come easily. It came from sitting with myself, again and again, especially on the days I felt lost. It came from making choices that felt aligned with my truth, even if they made no sense to others.

It came from learning to hear the whispers of my soul, those soft nudges that led me towards peace.

Peace, I realised, wasn't something I had to chase.

It was something I allowed.

It was found in the space I created within myself, once I stopped running from pain, and instead let it teach me.

For so long, my nervous system lived in survival. Braced for the next loss, the next betrayal, the next hard thing. But slowly, with every breath, every journaled tear, every healing session, I came back into my body.

I anchored into the *now*.

And in that presence, I began living in a new way, **aligned with my soul.**

Not with my wounds.

Not with my conditioning.

But with the truth of who I am, beneath it all.

It didn't mean life was always easy or perfect. But there was a clarity, a calm knowing, that no matter what came my way… I could meet it.

Not because I had control.

But because I had come home to myself.

Before I began this healing journey, I was always known as *the indecisive one* in the family. I'd be the last to choose what I wanted, the one who hesitated, doubted, and second-guessed herself until someone else made the decision for me. My sisters used to get vexed with me, "Just pick one!" they'd say. But I didn't trust myself. I didn't trust that what I wanted was right or allowed. And when I began to change, when I started listening to my own knowing and standing firmly in my decisions, it ruffled feathers. Not everyone welcomed the "healed" version of me. Because when we stop playing the roles others have grown used to, it can be uncomfortable for them. But it was never about pleasing them. It was about becoming me.

It's okay if some people in your life find the new you… different. They were simply familiar with the version of you that kept the peace, stayed small, or dimmed her light. The version who questioned herself, tiptoed around others' comfort, or carried what wasn't hers. When you begin to heal, to trust yourself, and to live more aligned with your soul, it can feel unfamiliar to those who knew you before. And that's okay. Not everyone is meant to walk beside the evolved version of you. Some will adjust. Some won't. But your growth isn't a betrayal. It's a homecoming.

🪶 Gentle Reflection: Coming Home to You

Take a quiet moment. Place your hand over your heart. Breathe slowly.

Ask yourself:

- *Where in my life am I still outsourcing my truth?*
- *What would it feel like to deeply trust myself today?*
- *When was the last time I felt truly at peace? What was I doing? Who was I with? How can I welcome more of that into my life now?*
- *Am I living in alignment with my soul—or someone else's expectations of me?*

There is no right answer here. Only what is real for you.

As you reflect, remember healing is not about becoming someone new. It's about remembering who you've always been. Underneath the fear, beneath the doubt, you are already whole. Welcome her home.

CHAPTER 9

Coming Home to Myself

There is a quiet kind of joy that comes when you realise you no longer need to search outside yourself for validation, love, or meaning. For most of my life, I was looking for permission, for belonging, for something to tell me I was enough. Or someone to tell me. But the deeper I journeyed through healing, the more I discovered that everything I was seeking had been inside me all along. I wasn't lost. I had just been disconnected.

Coming home to myself wasn't a dramatic moment; it was subtle and soft. It was learning to be present with myself. To enjoy my own company. To speak to myself with kindness. It was choosing rest without guilt. Saying "no" without apology. And allowing myself to be fully human, messy, radiant, healing, growing.

This chapter of my life feels like integration. The pain no longer defines me. The past no longer controls me. I honour what I've been through, but I no longer carry it. I've come home to the truth of who I am, a soul in a human body, here to experience love, connection, and meaning.

Coming home to yourself is the deepest form of self-love. It's remembering that you are already whole, already enough, already worthy. You always were.

As I journeyed deeper into healing, I began to notice something that felt almost magical, the subtle but constant presence of divine guidance. It started with the tiniest whispers, the synchronistic events that seemed too perfect to be coincidence. A random song on the radio that spoke directly to my heart, a chance encounter with someone who had the exact wisdom I needed at that moment, the way the universe seemed to line up events in my favour. At first, I questioned these experiences, wondering if I was reading too much into them. But the more I leaned into my trust, the more these moments became undeniable.

The most striking sign for me came in the form of white feathers and robins. At first, it felt like a coincidence, but then I started to see them everywhere, at the most crucial times. A white feather fluttering at my feet during a particularly heavy moment of grief, or a robin appearing right after I had asked for clarity in a prayer. These small but powerful signs began to remind me that I was not alone, that I was being held and supported every step of the way.

As someone who was never overly religious, I found this connection to the divine startling at first. But it also felt incredibly liberating. I was awakening to the fact that God, the Universe, or whatever higher power you connect with, is not a distant, abstract force. It's alive in every moment, in every breath, in every leaf that falls, and every bird that sings. God wasn't outside of me, looking in; God was within me, all around me, woven into the very fabric of my life. This realization deepened my faith and strengthened my trust in the process.

Reflection to Connect with Your Own Divine Guidance:

Take a moment to reflect on the signs and synchronicities in your own life. Can you recall a time when you felt a subtle pull or a divine nudge that led you to exactly what you needed? Perhaps a song, a chance meeting, or a seemingly random event that now feels like a message just for you?

Close your eyes and place your hands over your heart. Invite your higher self or any spiritual guides you resonate with to come close. Ask for guidance, whether it's clarity, comfort, or direction, and trust that the answers will come in ways that are meaningful to you. Open yourself to the quiet whispers and gentle signs the Universe is offering.

CHAPTER 10

The Divine in the Everyday

As I moved further along my healing journey, something profound began to shift within me. I had always sought divine experiences in the grand and the extraordinary, grand moments of prayer, rituals, and the occasional signs from the universe. But the more I healed, the more I realized that the divine isn't just in the moments of brilliance or in life-altering experiences. It's everywhere.

It's in the quiet morning light as it dances across the kitchen counter. It's in the laughter of my children; in the way their energy fills a room and makes my heart expand. It's in the simple act of breathing deeply, feeling the air fill my lungs, and knowing that each breath is a gift. These once ordinary moments began to hold so much meaning, as I saw them through the lens of my spiritual awakening.

I realized that the divine doesn't need to be sought out in faraway places or profound ceremonies. It's woven into the fabric of life, in the mundane and the miraculous alike. Every interaction, every feeling, every step on my path is infused with the divine. Whether it's a mundane errand, a quiet moment with my family, or an unexpected burst of inspiration during a meditation, these are all sacred moments.

The truth is, I had been living with a sense of separation. I thought I had to reach or strive for divinity, but now I see it was always right here with me, in the present. It's in the challenges, the struggles, and the victories, too. Every experience holds the potential for divine connection, if we are open enough to see it.

One of the most beautiful lessons I've learned is that when we allow ourselves to be present in the now, when we let go of expectations of what we think life should be, we open ourselves to the divine unfolding in the present moment. The universe is constantly speaking to us, not just in the grand events, but in the tiny details, the way the sun breaks through the clouds or the sound of rain against the window.

Healing, I've learned, is not just about changing the past or waiting for a grand moment of enlightenment, it's about waking up to the sacredness of the present. It's about feeling the connection with God, the universe, and the world around you in every moment. We don't need to wait for something big to happen to experience the divine. It's here, now, in every breath, every touch, every glance.

Reflection: Connect with the Divine in Your Everyday Life:

Take a moment to reflect on the simple moments in your day that you can now see as sacred. How can you begin to recognize the divine in the ordinary? Maybe it's the way the wind feels on your skin, the way your loved ones look at you with love, or the sensation of your feet connecting with the earth.

Find a quiet space and close your eyes. Take a few deep breaths and bring your awareness to the present moment. What do you feel?

What do you hear? What do you see around you? As you breathe in, invite the divine to be with you in this moment. Let go of expectations and allow yourself to feel connected to everything around you. Trust that you are not separate from the divine, you are part of it, and it is part of you.

As my connection to the divine deepened, I began to notice the subtle synchronicities that were unfolding in my life. At first, I thought they were mere coincidences—small, unimportant happenings that anyone could dismiss. But then, as I paid closer attention, I realized that these synchronicities were too aligned to be just chance.

I started seeing signs from the universe and from God in the most unexpected places. White feathers—seemingly insignificant, floating in places I least expected, like in my path when I was out for a walk, or on my kitchen counter. These feathers became a reminder that I was being guided, that I was never alone on my journey.

Robins, too, began to show up at the most serendipitous times. These little birds, so bright and full of life, seemed to appear out of nowhere, perched on a nearby fence or hopping along the ground when I needed to feel reassurance. Their presence became my signal that I was on the right path, that I was loved, and that I was supported by something greater than myself.

It wasn't just about these physical signs, though. It was the feeling that came with them—a deep sense of peace that washed over me. It was as if the universe itself was sending me a quiet message, reminding me that I was part of something larger, something eternal. The presence of God, I realized, wasn't just in the big moments of my life, but in these small, quiet signs that would often go unnoticed if I wasn't paying attention.

What I learned was that synchronicities are the universe's way of showing you that you are aligned with your higher purpose. They're like gentle nudges that guide you when you need it most. And the more I healed, the more I opened myself up to these synchronicities, knowing that they were reminders that I was being guided, that I was on the right path.

It wasn't always easy to trust in these signs. There were times when doubt would creep in, and I would question whether these were just my imagination or wishful thinking. But the more I leaned into the divine presence that I felt, the more I realized that the universe speaks to us in ways that are beyond our comprehension. The signs, the synchronicities, they were part of a larger plan, and I was in tune with it, whether I fully understood it or not.

Reflection: Recognizing the Divine Signs in Your Life:

Take a moment to reflect on any signs or synchronicities that have appeared in your life. Have you ever experienced a moment where something seemed too perfectly timed to be a coincidence? Maybe you've seen a white feather, noticed a robin, or felt a sudden, inexplicable sense of peace during a challenging time.

Take a deep breath and sit quietly. Ask yourself: How do these signs make you feel? Do they bring you a sense of comfort? Do they remind you that you are supported? Allow yourself to trust that the divine is always with you, speaking through the small, meaningful moments of your life.

By acknowledging these small signs, we can strengthen our connection to God and the universe. It's like a conversation between our souls and the divine. And when we open ourselves up to recognizing them, we start to see the world around us as a tapestry woven with love, guidance, and synchronicity.

As I continued to surrender to the divine flow of life, I found myself more attuned to the invisible forces that surrounded me. What I once considered mere coincidences began to feel like divine interventions, gentle reminders that God was always by my side, supporting me even in my darkest moments.

During the toughest parts of my healing journey, when I questioned my worth, my path, or whether I would ever truly heal, the presence of God and the archangels became undeniable. I was never alone in my suffering. It was as if I could feel a hand on my shoulder, an unseen force guiding me through the storm. This wasn't something I had ever truly understood before, and certainly not in the depth I did now.

I didn't grow up with a strong religious foundation. In fact, spirituality always felt like a foreign concept to me. I never imagined that my connection to God would evolve into something so intimate, so personal. Yet, here I was, in the midst of my grief and healing, finding solace in my faith in a way I had never experienced before. The more I allowed myself to open up to this connection, the more I felt my life shift.

The archangels, too, seemed to step into my life at just the right moments, offering their guidance and protection. Archangel Michael, the protector, became a constant source of strength for me. During times of fear or uncertainty, I would silently call on him, asking for courage and protection. His presence was calming, and I could feel the weight of my fears lift when I surrendered to his guidance.

Archangel Raphael, the healer, was another constant companion on my journey. When I felt physically or emotionally drained, I would ask for his healing energy to flow through me. It wasn't always immediate, but slowly, over time, I began to notice shifts within my body and mind. The energy of the archangels worked in ways that were subtle but powerful. They showed me that healing was a process, and though it wasn't always linear, it was always happening in its own time.

God, the archangels, and the synchronicities weren't something separate from me; they were a part of me, helping me align with my highest purpose. They were a reminder that I wasn't just a human going through life, but a soul on a sacred journey, guided by divine light. This realization gave me comfort and peace. It helped me trust that no matter what happened, I was never truly alone.

Reflection: Opening to Divine Guidance and Support:

Take a moment to reflect on your own spiritual path. Have you ever felt the presence of a higher power in your life? Maybe through signs, through a sense of peace, or through a gentle whisper of guidance?

Think about the times in your life when you've felt lost, afraid, or uncertain. How did you navigate through those moments? Did you sense a guiding hand, a sign that you were supported?

Allow yourself to tune into that energy now. Whether you believe in God, the universe, or a higher power, allow yourself to feel the comfort of knowing that you are never alone.

Take a deep breath, and in this moment, trust that you are always held in divine love.

As I look back now, I realize how deeply this trust in God and the angels has shaped my healing journey. It hasn't always been easy to let go of control, to trust in something I couldn't see with my physical eyes, but it has been one of the most transformative aspects of my life. The more I allowed myself to trust in the divine, the more aligned I felt with my soul's purpose, and the more peace I found within myself.

We are all being guided, even when we don't know it. Whether it's through a white feather, a robin, or a whisper in our hearts, the divine is always speaking to us. Learning to listen to these messages, to trust in the signs, and to open ourselves to the guidance of the angels and God, can lead us to a place of deep peace and alignment.

As you continue on your healing journey, I invite you to stay open to the divine. Trust that everything you need is already within you, and that you are never alone. Allow the synchronicities and signs to be your guide, as you move forward in faith, peace, and love.

CHAPTER 11

The Gift of Motherhood – My Why

Becoming a mother shifted something deep inside me. It was as though I suddenly became fully aware of the importance of what I was doing, not just in the moment, but in the bigger picture. I realized that my journey of healing wasn't just for me. It was for them, my children. They became my greatest motivators, the driving force behind every choice I made to heal, grow, and evolve.

Before they came into my life, I was navigating my own journey of healing, but motherhood brought a deeper sense of purpose. They were watching me, feeling my energy, and learning from me every single day. The realization that everything I did had the potential to shape their experiences, beliefs, and the way they saw the world was both empowering and humbling.

Every choice I made to heal, to grow, to release old wounds, became more than just an act of self-care. It became a way to enrich their lives, to give them the gift of emotional well-being, and to show them the power of resilience, compassion, and self-love.

They didn't ask for this. They didn't ask for me to heal or change. But the reality is, our children are constantly absorbing the energy we put out. They feel our emotions, our struggles, and our victories. And as much as I wanted to protect them from any pain, I also knew that the best way to protect them was to heal myself, to break the cycles of pain and trauma that had been passed down through generations.

My children became my mirror. They reflected back to me everything I needed to heal, everything I needed to let go of. Their pure, unconditional love reminded me of the importance of healing the inner child, of forgiving myself for past mistakes, and of stepping into my power as a mother and as a woman.

They are my greatest teachers. They've taught me patience, humility, and grace. They've shown me the true meaning of unconditional love. Every time I look at them, I am reminded of why I do this work, the deep desire to enrich their experience in life, to help them feel safe, loved, and empowered.

As much as I wanted to be the "perfect mother", whatever that is, I had to learn to let go of that ideal. I had to release the pressure I put on myself to always get it right. I realized that the best gift I could give them was not perfection, but authenticity. Showing them that it's okay to be human, to make mistakes, and to heal along the way.

Reflection: Your Children as Teachers of Healing

Take a moment to reflect on your relationship with your children or the children in your life. How have they inspired or motivated you on your own healing journey?

Think about how your energy, your emotions, and your actions influence their lives. In what ways can you show them the power of healing, self-compassion, and resilience?

What can you do today to enrich their experience in life, to give them the tools they need to feel loved, seen, and heard?

The Gift of Healing for Them

It's easy to think of healing as a personal journey, but the truth is, it affects everyone around us. Our healing journey isn't just about us; it's about breaking generational patterns, transforming our family's energy, and giving our children a different experience than the one we had.

Every time I release an old belief, heal a past wound, or forgive myself; I am not only healing myself but also healing the future generations. I am creating a space for my children to grow into the healthiest, happiest versions of themselves. I am setting the stage for them to live a life filled with love, empowerment, and peace.

In my heart, I know this is the greatest gift I could ever give them.

The Lights of My Life – Grace, Katie, and Joseph

Grace, my first born, the one who made me a mother. I am often saddened when I think of the time you came into the world. It was such a turbulent season in my life. We were waiting for my father to pass, and I was caught in the waves of anticipatory grief and all the emotional storms that followed. My moods were erratic, my pain deep and often unspoken. And yet, you were there, steady, beautiful, and full of light. Please know, my darling, you are the love of my life.

My *saving grace*. You were born in chaos, but you brought with you a quiet strength that has grounded me ever since.

Katie Tess Mannion. My rainbow baby. Tess, your name is a tribute to my grandmother, a woman who was both wildly loving and fiercely alive. You were born on a sunny Saturday afternoon into a room overflowing with love, excitement, and hope. You were the light that followed the storm, and you've shown us a softness, a deep sensitivity none of us had known before. You are pure sunshine. I wouldn't change a single thing about you, you are, to me, the very epitome of perfection. We love you beyond words.

And my Joey. My son, my son, my son. You are my pride and joy. The moment they placed you in my arms, I knew our family was complete. You are the son I never knew I needed, the moon and stars in my night sky. A true gift from God. The depth of feeling I hold for you is beyond words. I can't even begin to explain the love I have for you, it's immeasurable, infinite, and divine.

To Grace, Katie, and Joseph. *I love you to the moon and back again.* You are my purpose, my light, my greatest blessings. Everything I have healed, everything I have built, everything I continue to do in this life, is for you.

Reflection: A Mother's Heart

Being a mother is not just about giving life, it's about being willing to grow, to evolve, and to break generational cycles so our children don't have to carry what we once did. It's about learning to forgive ourselves for what we didn't know then and showing up each day with a heart that tries again. Healing as a mother is one of the bravest acts of love. It is choosing to be present, even when it hurts. Choosing to feel, even when it's uncomfortable. And choosing to rise, not just for ourselves, but for those little eyes watching and hearts depending on us.

Your children will know love, not because life is perfect, but because you chose to heal.

Journaling Prompt:

Take a quiet moment with your journal and ask yourself:

- *What parts of my healing have been inspired by my children?*
- *What lessons do I hope they learn by witnessing my growth?*
- *Is there anything I want to forgive myself for as a mother?*
- *What is one intention I can set today that will enrich their experience of life through my love?*

Let your answers come softly, like a conversation between your soul and the souls of your children.

A Mother's Prayer

Dear God,

Thank you for the gift of motherhood.

Thank you for the little souls who chose me,

even before I knew who I truly was.

Help me to be gentle—with them and with myself.

Guide me to love them in a way that frees them,

not in a way that binds them.

Show me how to listen—not just with my ears,

but with my whole heart.

And when I fall short,

remind me that even in my imperfections,

I am enough.

Let my healing be their foundation,

and let my love be their home.

Amen.

Affirmation:

I am a healing mother, a safe place, a guiding light.

Through my love, my children will know peace, strength, and the beauty of being wholly themselves.

CHAPTER 12

Never Alone – Wings of Light

For so long, I walked through life feeling disconnected. Not just from others, but from something bigger, something I couldn't name but longed for with every fibre of my being. I didn't grow up religious. God was a distant concept, a figure confined to books and ceremonies. But in the midst of my deepest pain, when I fell to my knees and my soul cracked wide open, I found something real. Something gentle. Something powerful.

God didn't come to me with thunder or lightning. He came in whispers. In quiet moments. In feathers left on windowsills. In robins that lingered longer than they should. In the perfect song at the perfect time. And most of all, in the deep knowing that I was never truly alone.

During the times when grief hollowed me out, when the world felt too heavy to carry, the Archangels surrounded me like a divine team of love and light. I didn't always know who I was calling on at first, but over time I began to feel their presence so clearly.

Archangel Michael, with his sword of truth, helped me cut the energetic cords that bound me to shame, guilt, and old versions of myself. He gave me courage when I felt too broken to begin again.

Archangel Raphael, the healer, placed his emerald light over my heart, helping me release pain stored in the body, grief that had nowhere to go until I finally let it move through me.

Archangel Gabriel, the messenger, stirred my voice and gave me the strength to speak my truth, first in private whispers, then in the pages of my journal, and now out loud in this book.

Archangel Uriel, the illuminator, brought clarity when I stood at crossroads. He helped me trust that even when I couldn't see the path, it was unfolding beneath my feet with divine precision.

It was after my pregnancy loss that I was introduced to the Archangels in a way that felt real and personal. My brother, in his own quiet and thoughtful way, gifted me a deck of Archangel oracle cards. I don't even think he knew what that gesture would come to mean for me. At the time, I was lost in grief, swimming in a silence that no one seemed able to reach. But when I held those cards in my hands, something shifted. For the first time, I felt like I wasn't alone in my pain.

Each card became a doorway to comfort. Messages from Michael, Raphael, Gabriel, Uriel, and others felt like little beams of hope sent directly from the heavens. I would sit in silence, shuffle gently, and ask for guidance. And the words I pulled would land with such precision, it often moved me to tears. It was like having an invisible circle of loving support around me, whispering: *We see you. We're here. You are not alone.*

That deck opened a sacred line of communication. It connected me to something ancient, something holy, something that reminded me I was cradled even when I couldn't feel it. The Archangels didn't take away my pain, but they helped me carry it. They helped me transform it. And slowly, I began to heal, not just my heart, but my faith too.

And through it all, God's presence was steady. Not judging. Not punishing. Just being. Just loving. I began to see God not as someone to fear, but as someone I was already part of. I saw God in the way sunlight danced through the trees. I felt Him in the sacred silence of early morning. I heard Him in the laughter of my children, in the wind, and in my own breath.

Synchronicities became my conversation with the Divine. Numbers repeating. Names whispered in dreams. Perfect moments arranged in ways no human hand could plan. They were reminders: "I'm with you. Keep going."

✧ Reflection: Wings of Light
A Whisper from the Angels

Close your eyes and take a few deep breaths. Place your hands over your heart. Feel the rise and fall of your chest as you breathe in peace… and exhale anything heavy.

Now, imagine yourself standing in a golden light. It's warm, soft, and safe. You're not alone here. All around you are beings of light, glorious, radiant Archangels. They form a circle around you, their energy calm, powerful, and full of love.

You might sense **Archangel Michael** behind you, wrapping you in a deep blue cloak of protection.

Archangel Raphael places his emerald green hands gently on your shoulders, sending healing into every cell of your body.

To your left, **Archangel Gabriel** leans in, whispering divine truth into your ear reminding you of your voice, your purpose, your light.

And before you, **Archangel Uriel** lights your path with golden wisdom, reminding you that you are never lost.

Take a moment here. Let yourself receive. You don't need to do anything or be anyone else. Just allow.

If there's something on your heart that you've been carrying, silently ask the angels for support.

Breathe in: *"I am divinely supported."*

Breathe out: *"I am never alone."*

✧ Journal Prompt:

- Have you ever felt a presence guiding or supporting you when you needed it most?
- What message do you think the Archangels would offer you right now?
- If you could surrender one worry, what would it be?

CHAPTER 13

Whispers of the Divine

There comes a point on every healing journey where the signs become too clear to ignore. A feather on the ground in the exact place you were about to give up. A robin at your window when you're deep in grief. A perfectly timed song, number, or encounter that speaks directly to your soul. Some would call these coincidences. But I came to understand them as whispers, divine messages, gently guiding me home.

In the quiet moments, in the ordinary days, I started to *see*. I began to recognise that I was never truly alone. That something much bigger than me had always been orchestrating my healing, even when I couldn't see the path ahead.

It started slowly, noticing repeating numbers like 11:11 or 444. White feathers would appear in the most unusual places, in the car, on the bathroom floor, in my children's bedrooms. The most bizarre feather we encountered was Christmas eve, 2024, my husband and I were setting up the sitting room before bed with all the kids' Christmas presents and just before we started, we both noticed a white feather in the middle of the sitting room. My father's favourite time of year was Christmas and he loved nothing more than getting the sitting room ready for the grandchildren on Christmas eve night. I know this was a sign. I know this was him, telling me that I wasn't alone, even though I really felt it that Christmas. I just missed that unconditional love that only he could give me.

And then the robins… they seemed to show up just when I needed a reminder that I was being watched over. Every time I doubted myself, a little, red-breasted robin would perch nearby, as if to say, "Keep going. You're doing just fine."

I didn't grow up deeply religious, and yet, this connection to God — to *my* understanding of God, became one of the most grounding and empowering parts of my healing. I realised that God was never far away. Not in the sky or in some distant heaven, but in *everything*. In the laughter of my children, the strength in my hands during a healing session, the stillness of nature, the warmth of the sun. God was in my breath. God was in me.

I began to co-create with life. I no longer felt like a victim of circumstance or a prisoner of grief. I was a divine being, deeply connected to the rhythm of the Universe. And when I fully opened my heart to that, when I began to *trust* that life was always working *for* me, not against me, everything changed.

Now, when I see the feathers, the robins, the signs and synchronicities, I smile. They are not just symbols of reassurance. They are sacred reminders that the veil between this world and the next is thinner than we think. That love never dies. And that guidance is always available when we open our hearts and ask to receive it.

EPILOGUE

And so, I Whisper Back

There was a time I believed that healing meant fixing myself.
That if I could just *try harder, do more, be better*, I would feel whole again.

But healing doesn't ask us to become someone new.

It gently invites us to remember who we were before the world told us who to be.

Grief cracked me open. Loss unravelled me.

But in that unravelling, I found something sacred: **my truth**.

I walked through the darkness. I sat in silence. I felt the ache of what had been and the hope of what might still come.

I wept. I raged. I prayed.

And through it all, I was held. I just didn't know it at the time.

Looking back now, I see the threads that wove it all together.

The whispers that guided me home.

The feathers, the robins, the synchronicities.

The way Grace, Katie, and Joseph became mirrors of the divine reminding me that love is the greatest teacher of all.

To the one reading this:

You are not broken. You are becoming.

There is wisdom in your wounds, and there is strength in your softness.

You don't need to have all the answers to take the next step.

You just need to trust the whisper that says,

"Keep going."

May you walk gently with your past.

May you honour the child within you.

May you make peace with your story.

And may you always remember, **you are never alone**.

There is a light within you that nothing can extinguish.

There is a soul within you that knows the way home.

And there are whispers, always whispers, reminding you…

You are loved.

You are guided.

You are enough.

Now and always.

A Prayer for Healing and Hope

Divine Source,

May your light surround this soul with gentle peace,

May your love wash over them like a healing river,

and may your whispers guide them on the path to wholeness.

I pray that they find courage in the silence,

strength in the softness,

and grace in every step they take.

Let them remember that they are whole, even in their brokenness,

and that every tear is a seed of transformation.

Grant them the wisdom to listen to their heart,

the clarity to see the light in the darkest of times,

and the peace to rest in the knowing that they are never alone.

May their soul find its way home,

and may love be the light that always leads them forward.

Amen.

A Blessing for the Journey Ahead

May you be blessed with the courage to walk your path,

with the strength to face whatever comes your way,

and with the peace that comes from surrendering to your soul's wisdom.

May you release what no longer serves you,

and embrace the beauty of the life that is unfolding before you.

May your heart be a vessel for compassion,

and may your soul be a beacon of love,

shining brightly for all who cross your path.

As you continue your journey, may you always be guided by light,

wrapped in love,

and held in grace.

And may you never forget

you are enough,

you are loved,

you are divinely supported.

Go find peace, dear soul, and may the whispers of your heart always lead you home.

Next Steps

No doubt reading this book has brought some emotions and struggles to the surface. You might feel a little lost or unsure about how to move forward, and that's completely natural. That's why I've shared my story, along with journal prompts, reflections, and meditations, to offer you tools that can guide you on your path.

But healing is a deeply personal process, and sometimes we all need a little extra support. If you feel that additional guidance could help you, I'd love you to reach out to me at evelyn_shine@hotmail.com or alternatively contact **Eriu Energy Healing.** I offer a space where you can access further resources or connect directly with me for personalised support on your healing journey.

Be kind to yourself as you move forward, and know that help is here when you need it. - Evelyn

www.ingramcontent.com/pod-product-compliance
Lightning Source LLC
Chambersburg PA
CBHW061234070526
44584CB00030B/4119